THE POWER OF FAITH AFFIRMATIONS

Speak Faith, Create New Realities

PASTOR (DR.) ENIS OLORUNNIPA
AND DR. MERCY OLORUNNIPA

ISBN: 978-1-960764-87-4 (sc)
ISBN: 978-1-960764-88-1 (hc)
ISBN: 978-1-960764-90-4 (eBook)

Write and Release
PUBLISHING

www.writeandreleasepublishing.com

TABLE OF CONTENTS

FOREWORD

Welcome to the journey of transformation through the power of affirmations. We are the Empyrean Couple and as a family, we have witnessed firsthand the remarkable impact of the spoken word of faith every aspect of our lives. Every success we have achieved has been directly tied to our faith affirmations - our success in ministry, sound health, a godly marriage, our pregnancy journey, our financial transformation, successes in businesses, all our houses, cars, jobs, residency status and more.

We began to learn about affirmations when we joined the ministry of our Man of God, Father, Life Coach, and the President of Loveworld Inc., Reverend Dr Chris Oyakhilome DSc DSc DD. All we know about affirmations, he taught us. And for this and many other reasons, we are eternally grateful to him. We are also blessed to be under the direct leadership of our Father, Highly Esteemed Regional Pastor and member of the Central Executive Council of Loveworld Inc., Reverend Ken Oyakhilome, one whose liquid love, audacious faith and bold affirmations have literally transformed our life and ministry.

In the pages of this book, we invite you to embark on a voyage of self-discovery and manifestation. Together, we have seen the impossible become possible, the unimaginable become reality. Through unwavering faith in our Lord Jesus Christ and affirmations rooted in the word of God, we have not only achieved but exceeded what many deemed unattainable.

What is it that you desire? Speak it into existence with faith and conviction. As you delve into the principles outlined in this book, you will discover the transformative potential of your own words. Our testimonies stand as evidence that through faith affirmations, anything is possible.

Join us as we unravel the secrets to unlocking your fullest potential and embracing a life filled with abundance, purpose, and fulfillment. The journey begins here, within the pages of this book, and extends far beyond, into the realm of infinite possibilities.

With unwavering belief and boundless optimism,

Pastor (Dr) Enis and Dr Mercy Olorunnipa

Chapter 1:

INTRODUCTION - UNDERSTANDING AFFIRMATIONS

Affirmation can be defined as the act of affirming a statement of the existence or truth of something; assertion. It is the assertion that something exists or is true.

Life is Spiritual

The spiritual controls the physical

There are those who subject themselves to the tutelage of the body, others that of the mind but pay little or no attention to the tutelage of the spirit.

God chose the foolish things of this world (for example, speaking/words) to confound the wise.

Weymouth New Testament Translation puts it beautifully

"But God has chosen the things which the world regards as foolish, in order to put its wise men to shame; and God has chosen the things which the world regards as destitute of influence, in order to put its powerful things to shame" - 1 Corinthians 1:27

Just like speaking in tongues, there are those who consider the topic of affirmations as unimportant. Such people are not different from Esau in the Bible whom the Bible calls profane because he undervalued, denigrated and had little or no regard for spiritual things. He sold his birthright with words (Genesis 25:28-34) but thought it was just a light thing.

We love how the Good News Bible puts it in Hebrews 12:16 "Let no one become immoral or unspiritual like Esau, who for a single meal sold his rights as the older son."

This is how many people are, they are unspiritual like Esau and some are even proud of it yet life is spiritual.

Don't end up like Esau for the Bible says in Hebrews 12:17 AMP

For you know that later on, when he wanted [to regain title to] his inheritance of the blessing, he was rejected, for he found no opportunity for repentance [there was no way to repair what he had done, no chance to recall the choice he had made], even though he sought for it with [bitter] tears.

Chapter 2:

BIBLICAL BASIS OF AFFIRMATIONS

Joshua 1:8

This book of the law shall not depart out of thy mouth; but thou shalt meditate therein day and night, that thou mayest observe to do according to all that is written therein: for then thou shalt make thy way prosperous, and then thou shalt have good success.

Some misquote the verse above. It says this book of the law shall not depart out of thy mouth not thy mind. That's affirmation! And He tells you you'd have good success if you do this. Meaning with affirmations you can determine your success

Affirmation is akin to code programming

A web developer writes codes that become a functionality for the user. You write the code of your new job on your heart and if that code executed correctly, it will manifest as that new job.

Psalms 45:1 says "My heart is inditing a good matter: I speak of the things which I have made touching the king: my tongue is the pen of a ready writer."

The word inditing means composing. Just like you'd compose a song in your heart but then strikingly He says my tongue is a pen. You compose with your heart, you write with tongue that is, by talking. Amazing!

Chapter 3:

THE MECHANICS OF AFFIRMATIONS

The next question is where do you write?

According to the Berean Study Bible, 2 Corinthians 3:3 reads

"It is clear that you are a letter from Christ, the result of our ministry, written not with ink but with the Spirit of the living God, not on tablets of stone but on tablets of human hearts."

The answer to that question above is in this scripture. You write words on the tablet of your heart with your affirmation.

So here's the principle:

"You have to say to believe so that you can now say what you believe in order to receive what you decreed"

The above statement is a very powerful one. Everything you ever want to accomplish through affirmations has to be inked on your heart first through the same affirmations. You have to say it enough in meditation to believe it. Once you've caught it in your spirit (your heart) that is written it in your spirit with the permanent ink of your words/ declarations, now you are ready to bring it out of that same heart into manifestation.

Chapter 4:

BRINGING AFFIRMATIONS TO FRUITION

You find this principle in several scriptures:

Proverbs 4:23
Keep thy heart with all diligence; for out of it are the issues of life.

The word issues refers to everything you want in life; your health, that job, that success in your business, that property, your marriage, children, those souls you want to win, that contract, that money everything you desire in this life comes from your heart. But how did they get in there? Through your talking.

The word issues also means springs. That is why Jesus said in John 7:38 “He who believes in Me, as the Scripture has said, out of his heart will flow rivers (springs) of living water.”

So simply put, the springs of your finance, marriage, health, business etc that you have created within you will now come forth through the same speaking.

Chapter 5:

HOW TO BRING OUT MONEY WITH AFFIRMATIONS

You might ask, what is the purpose of speaking them forth again since they are already springs inside you, well it's because you want to see the manifestations of those springs outside you, they are inside you now but you also want them outside. So you can understand why a man can say I am rich even when his accounts read zero. It is because he has billions inside him, he has through affirmations made those huge deposits in his spirit so you cannot convince him otherwise.

How to bring out the billions

The Bible says in Luke 6:45.. "...For out of the abundance of the heart his mouth speaks" now that your heart is filled with the springs of your house, you have to speak again. There must be a direct connection between your heart and your mouth. You must have believed it enough in your heart first then you speak it forth. If you haven't believed it, it will not work. You are saying what you have already acquired in your spirit.

Remember that the words coming out of you are springs/rivers. So the Bible says in Ecclesiastes 11:3 "If the clouds be full of rain, they empty themselves upon the earth..."

Understand that there are different clouds of life. You can have your academic cloud that is, everything that has to do with your academics then your financial cloud, your career cloud, your ministry cloud, your marriage cloud, your business cloud etc.

So the Bible says if any of your clouds be full of rain, they empty themselves. Oh hallelujah! This is so stirring.. this just explains why somebody might say "I have been making declarations regarding "xyz" but it hasn't manifested yet but I know I got it in my spirit already. Well maybe the clouds are not yet full. That is not the time to stop talking and say well whatever will be will be. No no no. What if the clouds were 99% full already and required just 1% more from you. Listen there is no word that you speak that doesn't form rain in your cloud. Understand that there are no empty words. And something to point out here is that the same way you have it in the positive so do you in the negative. If somebody will say "I'm going crazy" long enough, it's just a matter of time, the cloud of his insanity will be full and rain insanity on him. So if the cloud of your billions is full enough, it will empty those billions back to you or if you felt sick in your body, it's time to fill your health cloud with more rain so that it pours health back on you.

Chapter 6:

THE POWER OF DIRECTED AFFIRMATIONS

The next thing you need to understand is that for affirmations to work, they need to be directed appropriately. The Bible says:

"For as the rain cometh down, and the snow from heaven, and returneth not thither, but watereth the earth, and maketh it bring forth and bud, that it may give seed to the sower, and bread to the eater: so shall my word be that goeth forth out of my mouth: it shall not return unto me void, but it shall accomplish that which I please, and it shall prosper in the thing whereto I sent it."

Isaiah 55:10-11 KJV

This is God Almighty speaking and this was exactly how creation came into being. This was how God Almighty created the heavens and the earth and everything in it including YOU. 1This same pattern we are expected to follow. Remember the Bible says "... as He is so are we in this world". Also in Eph 5:1 "Therefore be imitators of God, as beloved children." We are expected to copy our Heavenly Father that is, to do what he does. Do you want peace in your home? This is the answer you've been looking for. Just like our Heavenly Father, release peace from your mouth and direct it to your home. In other words, send peace to your home and just know that it will prosper in the thing whereto you sent it (Luke 10:5-6). This is why you can be in one country and effect changes in another country. When you use words, don't be vague, be clear, be specific. That's why as a parent, you might have sent your child to school in a different location far from home, rather than worry over your child, every day direct words of affirmations to your child in that place then you can be at rest because your words will not return to you void but shall accomplish what you please and prosper in the thing whereto you sent it. Do you have your file on the table of the immigration officer awaiting a decision? Or do you have your file in court or your contract on that desk amongst other competitors? Is your resume or application in that pool of applicants? Now you know what to do.. send words specifically to your file and say what should happen to that file/document of yours and it will happen just as you have said.

Chapter 7:

THE PRINCIPLE OF BELIEF AND SPEAKING

You believe and then you speak. Our Lord Jesus said in Mark 11:23:

"For verily I say unto you, That whosoever shall say unto this mountain, Be thou removed, and be thou cast into the sea; and shall not doubt in his heart, but shall believe that those things which he saith shall come to pass; he shall have whatsoever he saith."

The principle upon which this book was written is clearly stated in the above scripture: our Lord Jesus said, "if you say to believe then you shall say to have that is you will have what you said that you have believed." That's a very powerful statement; read it over and over till it makes sense to you.

Also in 2 Corinthians 4:13 NIV:

It is written: "I believed; therefore I have spoken." Since we have that same spirit of faith, we also believe and therefore speak.

In affirmation, be specific. Looking closely at Mark 11:23, you'd see another important principle of affirmation right there in the first part. Our Lord Jesus said, "whosoever shall say unto THIS mountain". Don't miss a powerful principle of affirmation right there; He said "THIS" mountain. It was a specific mountain, he didn't speak generically by saying "whosoever shall say unto any mountain" rather he was specific. It's akin to a scripture we read earlier in Isaiah 55:11 "...it shall prosper in the thing whereto I sent it." There is a definite thing (place, situation, person) whereto the word was sent.

Here's the principle, if it's not clear to you, it will not be clear to the situation. What you are saying has to be very clear to you. For you to withdraw money from your ATM card, you have to input a definite/specific pin. The pin has to be exact for the card to work. It is the same with affirmation. When you say "I receive money today", what does money mean to you? What do you mean by money? How much are you talking about and in what currency? You don't type money into the ATM when you go to withdraw, do you? Rather you input the specific amount and currency so do the same with affirmation. For instance, say "I receive $10,000 today".

Chapter 8:

THE TRANSFORMATION OF WORDS

Words change state. You already know that water exists in 3 states: vapour/gaseous, liquid, and solid. The same water in a certain form cannot be seen (gaseous), in another form, you can see it but you cannot hold it (liquid), but in its third state, you can see it and hold it (solid). Words function similarly to the illustration above.

When you start releasing those words about your car, it was in gaseous state, then it gets converted to liquid and finally solid, into that car that you can touch and ride in. When the water was in gaseous state, it wasn't less water than the solid state. The water already existed though may not have been seen but it's as real as its solid state. Many often give up at the gaseous state while some others at the liquid state but those who sustain their confessions/declarations/affirmations always have tangible results to hold unto.

Chapter 9:

LIVING A FULFILLING LIFE

How to live a long, prosperous, healthy, and fulfilled life:

1 Peter 3:10:

For the Scriptures say, “If you want to enjoy life and see many happy days, keep your tongue from speaking evil and your lips from telling lies.”

Proverbs 18:21 NLT:

The tongue can bring death or life; those who love to talk will reap the consequences.

Proverbs 6:2 NIV:

You have been trapped by what you said, ensnared by the words of your mouth.

The answer you need is right there with you. You know many times people go everywhere (except to themselves) either in person or online seeking solutions/answers yet the Bible says the answer you need is right there where you are, inside you. Where exactly? In your heart and in your mouth, in other words "in your believing and in your speaking". Romans 10:8 says "But what does it say? "The word is near you, in your mouth, and in your heart." That is, the word of faith which we proclaim." Reading it this way may not be as clear but the Aramaic Bible in Plain English puts it perfectly "But what does it say? "The answer is near your mouth and your heart." This is the word of the faith that we preach."

Don't speak idle words, lay premium on words. There are a few lines I want you to keep with you from this part of the book.

Say what you mean and mean what you say. If you put premium on words, words will put premium on you. If you value words, words will value you. If words don't mean much to you, they won't mean much to the situation.

Matthew 5:37 New American Bible:

Let your 'Yes' mean 'Yes,' and your 'No' mean 'No.' Anything more is from the evil one.

Our Lord Jesus said in Matthew 12:36:

"But I say unto you, That every idle word that men shall speak, they shall give account thereof in the day of judgment."

Chapter 10:

THE POWER OF RESPONSE

He said so that you may boldly say... There are those who read the Bible like a novel, a news blog, newspaper or some textbook but they are wrong. The Bible, the word of God is a person. When you read the word, He is speaking to you and you are expected to respond. Imagine if someone sent you a text message, a response is expected. If you keep receiving messages without response, you may soon stop receiving those messages. The way God expects us to respond to the word is reflected in Hebrews 13:5-6

"Let your conversation be without covetousness; and be content with such things as ye have: for he hath said, I will never leave thee, nor forsake thee. So that we may boldly say, The Lord is my helper, and I will not fear What man shall do unto me." The emphasis is on "...for he hath said, I will never leave thee, nor forsake thee. So that we may boldly say…" The reason our Lord Jesus sent you the text in John 16:33 "These things I have spoken unto you, that in me ye might have peace. In the world ye shall have tribulation: but be of good cheer; I have overcome the world." is so that you may boldly say "I have peace in Christ Jesus and I have overcome the world. There may be troubles and tribulations all around me but I remain cheerful because the Lord Jesus has overcome the world for me therefore I am more than a conqueror"

This the same principle the systems of the world copy. Your company has said your salary would be paid on the 30th of the month so you boldly say I'm getting paid by the end of the month. The pilot has said you would be landing by 5pm so that you may boldly say to your family I would be arriving by 5pm, the google map has said it would take you 35 minutes to arrive your destination so you can boldly say to your boss I will be there in 35 minutes. If you could trust the world's systems that much, how much more God? What has the word of God said concerning you so that you may boldly say? It's high time you discovered those truths.

The Bible says "When men are cast down, then thou shalt say, There is lifting up; and he shall save the humble person." Job 22:29 Many misread this scripture as "when men say there's a casting down..." No, that's not what the Bible says. The Bible says "when men are cast down...". Think about the economic situation of many nations and how men are cast down for lack of money, food, or even security. In such a situation, many people try to be humble by saying things to identify with the situation but God wants you to respond otherwise. Don't take sides with the poor economic situation, don't take sides with the "plandemic", don't take sides with men; rather take sides with the word. When you speak that way, you may be perceived as arrogant, proud, and even insensitive, but all of that doesn't matter. What matters is doing what God has said. So the next time someone is cast down around you, don't collapse into the same situation; rather, declare there's a lifting up because your declaration will not only make an impact on you but on the downcast. Just like the second part of that scripture said "...and he shall save the humble (downcast) person."

Chapter 11:

STAYING ON THE FENCE IS NOT AN OPTION

Staying on the fence is not an option. The weeds will still grow. There are those who are of the opinion that you don't have to speak. They take a neutral stand when it comes to affirmation, but they are wrong. Think about it this way: when you plant crops on the ground, those crops grow provided the conditions are right. However, if you leave the land fallow without planting anything, growth will still happen—not of crops (because you didn't plant anything), but of weeds. And what are weeds? They are wild plants growing where they are not wanted and in competition with cultivated plants. This, therefore, means where affirmations are not spoken, certain things might seem to be going right but unwanted things will still show up. Such people will experience an up and down life, inconsistent results. They win today and lose tomorrow, well today and sick tomorrow, having today and lacking tomorrow. Speaking empty/idle words also act like weeds, they produce an unstable life. Before wrapping up this part, I'd like to highlight the second part of the definition of weeds which is the fact that these wild plants can also show up even where the land is cultivated with plants and then be in competition with the cultivated plants. This gives the understanding that if you want to win consistently, you'd have to flood your life with affirmations in abundance not sparsely such that there's no room for weeds and if peradventure any weeds show up, you weed them out immediately with the sword of the spirit (rhema), that is the spoken word of God (affirmations)

Chapter 12:

THE WATER AND RICE EXPERIMENT (A LOVE/ HATE EXPERIMENT)

We recently watched some videos online that featured what is now known as the love and hate rice experiment. The idea comes from an original experiment done some years ago by a Japanese man called Dr. Masaru Emoto who did an experiment that featured putting water into different petri dishes, exposing the water to different words and emotions, and then freezing the water samples to see how the crystals of water had arranged themselves. The results showed that the crystals of water that had positive words like love and gratitude had frozen into beautiful crystals of water that looked like amazing snowflakes, while the water that had been exposed to hate had crystals that had frozen into no real structure and ended up looking like murky blobs of water.

Dr. Masaru Emoto created a similar experiment on rice a few years later which has been the experiment that many people online have tried to reproduce, where three jars are filled with water and rice and are sealed. The water being the key component and the rice a way of visibly seeing the results as it would absorb the water. Every day one jar labelled 'love' had people saying loving things to it, like: I love you, you are wonderful, I appreciate you, etc. Another jar marked 'hate' is spoken to in a horrible way: I hate you, you should die, you are horrible, etc. And the third jar is simply marked 'ignore' which is what people do with it. Many people have tried to recreate this experiment with not only rice but apples sliced in half, even strawberries and some with plants. With respect to the experiments, skeptics will always state that bacteria and other contaminants in the air are responsible for the results of what happens in these experiments but there is something interesting in the results that many people have reported.

In Dr. Masaru Emoto's experiment, and many others conducted online, the results showed that the rice (or apple/strawberry/plant) that heard lovely loving words was still in good condition after a few days/weeks, while the 'hate' rice was going moldy and bad. The rice that was ignored did not do so well either. With results like this, the only conclusion Dr. Masaru Emoto and others have is how powerful words are and how, if water can be so affected by words (and affects the things it's in contact with like the rice) then what effect do these words have on our own bodies which are made up of 60% to 70% water too?

Whether you agree the rice or water experiments are real or not, I really don't think it matters, although personally I do believe they are legitimate experiments and you can try it for yourself if you like. What really matters is that words are more powerful than we think. Words are powerful things, and the emotions that go with those words can have such an impact on one's health and well-being. We underestimate how powerful words are, how much they can affect us throughout our lives. Words have meanings. Many today still believe in the hateful or negative things they were told when they were younger. They find it hard to say something positive because they always feel unworthy, undeserving or unlovable. Yet the negative, derogatory, hateful comments come so easily to them and many with low confidence and self-esteem choose to say those negative words to themselves or even to others when lashing out. But nobody expects a child born into this world to hate themselves. Nobody wants to see a child cry, despair and feel unworthy of happiness and life. And if no child deserves that then why would they when they grow up. The fact is, no matter what has happened in your life, words are powerful. Negative words are filled with the power to make people doubt themselves, to make them feel unworthy and unlovable. But positive words have the power to heal those wounds, to make us feel worthy, happy, loved and excited to face the world we live in.

Chapter 13:

WORDS ARE SEEDS AND YOUR HEART IS THE FIELD

Words are seeds, and your heart is the field. Our Lord Jesus refers to words as seeds in Luke 8:11 KJV: Here, then, is the deeper meaning to my parable: The word of God is the seed that is sown into hearts.

From verse 12 to 15, the Lord distinguishes amongst different grounds of the heart. "The hard pathway represents the hard hearts of those who hear the word of God but the slanderer quickly snatches away what was sown in their hearts to keep them from believing and experiencing salvation. The seeds falling on gravel represents those who initially respond to the word with joy, but soon afterward, when a season of difficulty and harassment of the enemy comes to them, they wither and fall away, for they have no root in the truth and their faith is temporary. The seeds that fall into the weeds represent the hearts of those who hear the word of God but their growth is quickly choked off by their own anxious cares, the riches of this world, and the fleeting pleasures of this life. This is why they never become mature and fruitful. The seed that fell into good, fertile soil represents those lovers of truth who hear it deep within their hearts. They respond by clinging to the word, keeping it dear as they endure all things in faith. This is the seed that will one day bear much fruit in their lives." Luke 8:12-15 TPT

So the big question is what kind of soil is your heart? Is it a hard ground or a fertile one? Read the criteria to answer that question again in Luke 8:12-15 (in different translations).

Chapter 14:

THE CHINESE BAMBOO TREE

We heard about the story of the Chinese Bamboo Tree and we'd like to share it with you. A Chinese bamboo tree takes five years to grow. It has to be watered and fertilized in the ground where it has been planted every day. It doesn't break through the ground for five years. After five years, once it breaks through the ground, it will grow 90 feet tall in five weeks! The question is did the Chinese bamboo tree grow 90 feet tall in five weeks or in five years? The answer is obvious, it grows 90 feet tall in 5 years. If at any time that person stopped watering and fertilizing that tree, it would die in the ground. Some people do not have the patience to wait for the tree to grow so that growth is truncated and the tree never shows up. Affirmation is like that. Our man of God Pastor Chris would always say, "keep saying it, don't stop talking it". He'd also say "if you stick to the word, you'd come back with a testimony."

Many people have been watering and fertilizing their seeds (in ministry, business, career etc) for many, many years; maybe without visible results. Don't give up, don't feel discouraged and don't stop because you are closer than you think. Just like the bamboo tree, suddenly, your work, business, finance will grow and manifest. If you've been speaking/watering your seeds for 10 years without visible results, if you will not stop, when the results would manifest it will be the growth of 10 years. Hallelujah.

Chapter 15:

THE POWER OF "I AM"

Isaiah 33:24 Majority Standard Bible says, "And no resident of Zion will say, "I am sick." The people who dwell there will be forgiven of iniquity."

Who are the beneficiaries of this blessing today? God's children. Who are those dwelling in Zion today, anyone who is born again, the Christian. So the Bible says you shall not say "I am sick". Why does he say so? Because of where you are dwelling. The name of God is named upon them that dwell in Zion.

Now pay very close attention. Our God described himself to Moses as "I am" so "I am" is the name of God meaning God = I am and I am = God. So you see saying "I am sick" is equal to saying "God sick". The question then becomes "can God be sick?", the answer is No. So if God cannot be sick neither can you. Someone might say that God, I am a man. Well let me show you a few scriptures that might surprise you Psalms 82:6 "I said, 'You are "gods"; you are all sons of the Most High.'"Jesus answered them, Is it not written in your law, I said, Ye are gods? If he called them gods, unto whom the word of God came, and the scripture cannot be broken; say ye of him, whom the Father hath sanctified, and sent into the world, Thou blasphemest; because I said, I am the Son of God?" John 10:34-36 KJV.

Just in case you're still in doubt, Read 1 John 4:17 KJV "Herein is our love made perfect, that we may have boldness in the day of judgment: because as he is, so are we in this world."

He has made us just as He is. So now that you have been enlightened in the word, every time you use "I am" as referring to yourself also remember that you are referring to God because He has made you His representative here on earth. Therefore the next time you say "I am..." in a sentence, ensure to fill it with only things that are consistent with the nature and character of God. Lack is not consistent with God, neither is failure, confusion, death etc so "I am not broke" because "I am cannot be broke" rather I declare that "I am rich and wealthy" "I am healthy and full of life" "I am sound", "I am..." you can fill in the bracket.

Chapter 16:

THE SPIRITUAL CONTROLS THE PHYSICAL

The currency we spend in the realm of the spirit is words.

God created everything with words, He said it and saw it, that it was good in Genesis chapter 1 but it took the next chapter for those things that He already created in the spirit to manifest in the physical.

Anything you cannot see, you cannot have. Even if you got it you'd lose it, just a matter of time. You have to see it in the spirit first.

Heb 10:23 NLT Let us hold tightly without wavering to the hope we affirm, for God can be trusted to keep his promise. Heb 4:14 NIV Therefore, since we have a great high priest who has ascended into heaven, Jesus the Son of God, let us hold firmly to the faith we profess. 1 Tim 6:12 Fight the good fight of faith, lay hold on eternal life, whereunto thou art also called, and hast professed a good profession before many witnesses. Phil 1:6 That the communication of thy faith may become effectual by the acknowledging of every good thing which is in you in Christ Jesus.

Examples: The wife who said she'd die.

There's a story of a woman who died the same day her husband died. That's a very sad thing but the reality was that she spoke her death to reality. It was reported that one day while playing with her husband, he asked her "If I die today what would you do and the lady said "I'll die too that very day". So it had happened that her husband traveled and was involved in a fatal car accident, everyone else in the vehicle survived except her husband. When the woman heard about the loss of her husband, she said she would not believe until she saw his corpse with her eyes. So while she was being driven to accident site, another accident occurred and everyone in that vehicle survived except the lady. Why would such a thing happen to anyone you might ask? Well the answer is given in Proverbs 6:2 NIV "you have been trapped by what you said, ensnared by the words of your mouth." Her words had trapped her.

Here's another example of a different lady who had died and then the Angel of God appeared to her and instructed her to return to her body. That was definitely a miracle but the more powerful part was the reason the Angel gave her for that instruction. The Angel told her that she had spoken too much life to die and then told her she would have to retract all the life she has spoken but not only that speak as much death as she has spoken life to die. Praise God! The miracle happened and she returned to life. Her words brought her back to life because in Proverbs 18:21 Berean Standard Bible "Life and death are in the power of the tongue, and those who love it will eat its fruit." According to the 2 examples above, one chose life and the other chose death, choose life. The scripture says in Deuteronomy 30:19 "Today I have given you the choice between life and death, between blessings and curses. Now I call on heaven and earth to witness the choice you make. Oh, that you would choose life, so that you and your descendants might live!" Oh hallelujah.

Chapter 17:

YOUR SALVATION CAME BY WORDS

Even your very salvation came by words. For you to be a Christian, it happens by words.

Romans 10:9-10 "If you declare with your mouth, "Jesus is Lord," and believe in your heart that God raised him from the dead, you will be saved. For it is with your heart that you believe and are justified, and it is with your mouth that you profess your faith and are saved.

Maturity is measured in your affirmations.

James 3:2 CEV All of us do many wrong things. But if you can control your tongue, you are mature and able to control your whole body.

James 3:2 AMPC For we all stumble and sin in many ways. If anyone does not stumble in what he says [never saying the wrong thing], he is a perfect man [fully developed in character, without serious flaws], able to bridle his whole body and rein in his entire nature [taming his human faults and weaknesses].

Your tongue is your body thermostat.

A thermostat exerts control by switching heating or cooling devices on or off, or by regulating the flow of a heat transfer fluid as needed, to maintain the correct temperature.

The Bible says in James 3:2 CEV All of us do many wrong things. But if you can control your tongue, you are mature and able to control your whole body.

This above scripture means you use your tongue, your affirmations to control/regulate your body. With your affirmations you can switch off sickness in your body and turn on health, you can switch off failure and turn on success, you can switch off lack and turn on unending prosperity, the switch is right there with you. Use it as you will.

You know incantations?

Growing up we saw some movies where the actors used incantations to invoke spiritual powers to achieve supernatural results. Though mostly evil outcomes in those movies, what they do is actually a copy of the original. Incantations come from God and are to be used to achieve good results. If you want to learn more about incantations make sure you are a part of our community.

Chapter 18:

TRUTH VS. FACT

THE TRUTH VS THE FACT

Someone once defined 'fact' as a piece of information about circumstances that exist or events that have occurred. However, 'truth' is what the Word of God says about the same circumstances or events. The Word is truth (John 17:17); it is reality. Job 22:29 clearly shows the difference between the fact and the truth. It shows us that even though it's a fact that everything is hopeless and there's no sign that things are going to get better, we can still declare the truth of God and say, "We're lifted up everywhere." Hallelujah! It's very important that you realize the difference between fact and truth. Otherwise, you wouldn't know how to take yourself out of any undesirable situation using the principle of confession. For example, a man had an accident and the x-ray showed that his bone was broken. When he was told, he said, "No, the bone is not broken in

Jesus' Name!" There's a difference between denying the fact and denying fact the power to determine the circumstances of your existence. Affirmation is not the denial of fact but denying the fact, the ability, the right to control your existence "truth".

The Bible never told us to deny the fact of our situation; rather, it says we should proclaim, confess or affirm the truth of God's Word in the situation. It was a fact that the man's bones were broken, however, the truth says, "...by whose (Jesus') stripes ye were healed" (1 Peter 2:24). So, the man's declaration ought to have been: "By the stripes of Jesus Christ I am healed." Declaration of the truth activates the power of God causing the situation to conform to your declaration.

Therefore, refuse to be dominated by the facts of your situation, rather let the truth of God be your focus. Fill your ears, eyes, mouth and heart with it, so you can effect any change you desire in your life today.

Facts may not always be true. To better understand this, think about yourself and how many times you've been probably misjudged maybe at the way you looked at someone or spoke to someone. The fact was that you looked in that awkward way or spoke those words you're being accused of but the truth was that it was a misrepresentation of the thoughts and intents of your heart.

Chapter 19:

SPEAK FORTH YOUR BABY

We had to dedicate a chapter to childbearing not only because it's a topic that touches many people but because of our own personal experiences too. It took us longer than we expected to conceive but thank God for faith affirmations. We brought forth our baby through our faith affirmations, designed the pregnancy journey by faith affirmations and now sustaining our son through the same faith affirmations. You too can bring forth your baby. So many people have followed these same principles that we have shared and returned with testimonies. Your story will not be different. Irrespective of the medical conditions or other seemingly negative circumstances, you will have your babies. There is no hopeless situation with God. Remember the earth was without form and void but the spoken word of God changed the entire situation and brought creation into being.

We have an entire book titled “Pregnancy Affirmations” by Dr Mercy Olorunnipa which is highly recommended for any pregnant woman or aspiring mother. In that book, there are powerful affirmations for the first trimester, second trimester, third trimester and for delivery. Just to give you a snippet of the book, did you know our baby came out without “pushing”? When you hear such things, the Hebrew women in the Bible may come to your mind but we dare tell you that this experience was better than the Hebrew women. You too can achieve the same result through your faith affirmations. The book is available online and also in print so make sure to place your order(s) today. We also have videos on our different online platforms where we shared the full story of “The Biggest Secret of our Successful Pregnancy Journey”. Just search for “The Empyrean Couple” online and you will able to watch our mind blowing testimonies with real evidence in pictures and videos.

Chapter 20:

EVERYBODY AFFIRMS EVERY DAY

There is no one who doesn't believe in affirmation. The truth actually is that everybody affirms every day. When you say to your colleague at work "I'll see you tomorrow", that is affirmation. You believe in your heart that you will be at work tomorrow and then you vocalized it. When you say, I'll call you in 5 minutes, that's affirmation. So you see, as long as you speak every day, you actually affirm every day. Now it's time to get more intentional with words. Rather than just remain at the level of those spontaneous affirmations, you can be more deliberate now and use your words to create your today and your tomorrow, use affirmations to shape your life and destiny.

Chapter 21:

AFFIRMATIONS FOR FAMILY

1. My family is blessed and favored by the Lord.
2. Love and harmony abound in our home.
3. We communicate with understanding and kindness.
4. Each member of my family walks in God's purpose and destiny.
5. Our home is a sanctuary of peace and joy.
6. Every member of my family is an ambassador of the Kingdom of God, we represent Him wherever we are
7. God's wisdom guides our decisions as a family.
8. Our family is God's outstretched hand to a hurting world
9. Divine protection surrounds each member of my family.

10. Our family is a shining example of God's love to others.
11. We speak words of encouragement and affirmation over each other daily.
12. Unity and cooperation characterize our family relationships.
13. Forgiveness flows freely, fostering healing and restoration.
14. My family is a beacon of hope and encouragement to others.
15. We are grateful for the blessings of togetherness and unity in our family.

Chapter 22:

AFFIRMATIONS FOR MARRIAGE

1. My marriage is founded on the rock of Christ, unshakeable and enduring.
2. Beauty, praise and joy characterize our marriage.
3. We communicate openly and honestly, with grace and understanding.
4. God's peace reigns in our hearts and home, guarding our relationship.
5. marriage is a reflection of Christ's love for the Church.
6. We prioritize each other's needs and seek to serve one another selflessly.
7. Our union grows stronger with each passing day, deepening in intimacy and trust.
8. We face and win challenges together, united in purpose and resolve.

9. Our marriage is a testimony of God's faithfulness and grace.
10. We honor and cherish each other, celebrating the gift of marriage daily.
11. Our relationship is shielded from discord and strife by God's protective hand.
12. We speak words of affirmation and encouragement, building each other up.
13. Our commitment to one another is unwavering, rooted in covenant love.
14. We cultivate romance and passion, keeping the flame of love burning brightly.
15. Our marriage glorifies God and serves as a light to others, inspiring hope and restoration.

Chapter 23:

AFFIRMATIONS FOR BUSINESS

1. My business is established on godly principles and integrity.
2. Divine favor characterizes my business, opening doors of opportunity.
3. I operate with wisdom and discernment in all my business dealings.
4. God's provision flows abundantly, meeting every need of my business.
5. My business excels, prospers and thrives, bringing glory to God.
6. I attract loyal and trustworthy clients/customers who value my products/services.
7. Divine connections and partnerships are orchestrated for the advancement of my business.

8. I am a wise steward of the resources entrusted to me, sowing generously into Kingdom purposes.
9. Innovation and creativity are unleashed in my business, leading to persistent productivity.
10. God's guidance directs my steps, leading me to profitable opportunities.
11. I am a channel of blessing through my business, impacting lives, communities and nations.
12. My business is a platform for Kingdom expansion, spreading God's love and truth.
13. Financial abundance and prosperity overflow in my business, enabling me to be a blessing to others.
14. I walk in excellence and diligence, setting high standards in my industry.
15. My business is a vehicle for God's Kingdom agenda, bringing transformation to society.

Chapter 24:

AFFIRMATIONS FOR FINANCE

1. I am a steward of God's resources, managing my finances with wisdom and integrity.
2. Divine provision meets all my needs according to His riches in glory.
3. I walk in financial abundance and overflow, blessed to be a blessing.
4. God's favor characterizes my finances, opening doors of opportunity and increase.
5. I sow generously into the Kingdom of God, knowing that I reap bountifully.
6. My investments are prospered by the hand of God, yielding supernatural returns.
7. I do not owe rather I lend to nations; I am debt-free and live in financial abundance.
8. I am a wise steward of God's unlimited and incalculable resources.

9. Divine wisdom guides my financial decisions, leading me to walk daily in paths of prosperity.
10. My bank accounts are overflowing with money, I am a money farmer.
11. I function in and from the economy of heaven therefore I do not know when heat comes.
12. I bear fruits in my finances always, in and out of season I flourish.
13. I always have money - money to give, money to invest, money to save and money to spend.
14. I am empowered to create wealth and establish God's will in the earth.
15. My financial harvest is plentiful, and I am positioned to be a conduit of God's blessing to others.

Chapter 25:

AFFIRMATIONS FOR HEALTH

1. I walk in divine health and wholeness 24 hours every day.
2. I declare that every cell and organ in my body in vitalized by the Spirit of God.
3. I refuse to be sick because God lives in me and greater is He that is in me than he that is in the world.
4. I walk in divine strength and energy, equipped to fulfill my purpose.
5. Sickness and disease have no power over me; because I live in the name of the Lord Jesus.
6. I speak life and health to every part of my body, aligning with God's Word.
7. Divine immunity shields me from every form of illness and infirmity.
8. I refuse to be weak, because the Lord is my strength therefore I am strong even now.

9. I am fearfully and wonderfully made, designed for health and wholeness.
10. I cancel/neutralize every negative report concerning my health, standing on the truth of God's Word.
11. By the stripes of our Lord Jesus, I am healed and made whole, body, soul, and spirit (if you feel sick).
12. I nourish my body with wholesome food, stewarding my health wisely.
13. Divine life flows through me, rejuvenating and revitalizing every part of my being.
14. I declare that the life of God is at work in every fibre of my being, causing me to walk in divine health and vitality.
15. My body is the temple of the Holy Spirit, and I honor God with my body by maintaining optimal health and well-being.

Chapter 26:

AFFIRMATIONS FOR ACADEMICS

1. I have the mind of Christ, endowed with wisdom and understanding.
2. Divine insight and revelation guide me in my studies and learning.
3. I am diligent and disciplined in my academic pursuits, excelling in all areas.
4. God's favor characterizes my academic endeavors, opening doors of opportunity and success.
5. I am anointed to grasp and comprehend even the most challenging subjects.
6. Divine wisdom flows through me, enabling me to excel academically.
7. I am a quick learner, absorbing knowledge and information effortlessly.
8. God's Word is a lamp unto my feet and a light unto my path, illuminating my studies.

9. I approach every academic challenge with confidence and boldness, knowing that I am more than a conqueror.
10. I am focused and determined to achieve excellence in my academic pursuits.
11. Divine intelligence operates in me, surpassing human understanding.
12. I am destined for greatness, and nothing can hinder the fulfillment of God's purpose in my life.
13. I excel in my academics, achieving top grades and academic honors.
14. I am a diligent student, dedicated to maximizing my potential and talents.
15. My academic success glorifies God and serves as a testimony of His faithfulness and grace.

Chapter 27:

AFFIRMATIONS FOR JOB

1. I am positioned for success and advancement in my career/job.
2. Divine favor characterizes my life, opening doors of opportunity and promotion.
3. I excel in my job, demonstrating excellence and integrity in all my tasks.
4. I am recognized and appreciated for my contributions and commitment.
5. God's wisdom guides my decisions and actions in the workplace, leading to success and favor.
6. I am a valuable asset to my company/organization, bringing creativity and innovation to my role.
7. Divine connections and relationships are established for my professional growth and development.

8. I am empowered to overcome every challenge and obstacle in my job, emerging victorious.
9. My skills and talents are recognized and rewarded, leading to increased responsibility and influence.
10. I walk in confidence and boldness, knowing that God is with me in every aspect of my job.
11. I am a leader and influencer in my workplace, impacting others positively with my character and integrity.
12. I am prosperous and successful in my career/job, fulfilling my God-given purpose and destiny.
13. Divine opportunities for advancement and promotion are released to me, elevating me to new levels of success.
14. I am blessed in my work, experiencing divine favor and prosperity in all my endeavors.
15. My job/career is a platform for Kingdom impact, and I am positioned to make a difference in the lives of others.

Chapter 28:

AFFIRMATIONS FOR MINISTRY

1. I am called and anointed by God for ministry, equipped with His power and authority.
2. Divine opportunities to minister and serve abound in my life, and I walk in obedience to God's leading.
3. I am a vessel of honor, sanctified and prepared for every good work in the Kingdom.
4. God's Word is my foundation and guide in ministry, and I declare it with boldness and conviction.
5. Signs, wonders, and miracles characterize my ministry, confirming the Word with power.
6. My ministry is pleasing to God, it brings glory to His name always.
7. Divine connections and divine appointments are orchestrated for the advancement of God's Kingdom through my ministry.

8. I walk in humility and dependence on the Holy Spirit, allowing Him to lead and guide me in ministry.
9. Souls are saved, lives are transformed, and captives are set free through my ministry.
10. I am a faithful steward of God's Word and gifts, using them to build up the body of Christ and edify believers.
11. I walk in divine protection always as I carry out my work of ministry diligently.
12. I am anointed to preach the Gospel with boldness and clarity, making disciples of all nations.
13. My ministry bears fruit that remains, impacting generations for the Kingdom of God.
14. I am a channel of God's love and grace, ministering to the brokenhearted and downtrodden.
15. My ministry brings glory and honor to God, advancing His Kingdom agenda on earth.

Chapter 29:

AFFIRMATIONS FOR CHILDREN

1. My children are a heritage and blessing from the Lord, fearfully and wonderfully made.
2. Divine protection surrounds my children, shielding them from all harm and danger.
3. They walk in obedience and wisdom, honoring God in all their ways.
4. God's favor characters the lives of my children, opening doors of opportunity and success.
5. They are taught by the Lord, and great is their peace and prosperity.
6. My children excel academically, intellectually, and creatively, demonstrating God's excellence in their lives.
7. They are filled with the Holy Spirit, walking in love, joy, and peace.

8. The Lord is their portion therefore they walk in divine health and wholeness, and sickness and disease have no power over them.
9. My children are leaders and influencers in their generation, impacting the world for Christ. My ministry brings glory and honor to God, advancing His Kingdom agenda on earth.
10. They have a heart for God and His Kingdom, serving others with compassion and humility.
11. Divine wisdom guides their decisions and choices, leading them in paths of righteousness.
12. My children are blessed with godly friendships and relationships that inspire them more and more in the things of God.
13. All my children are relevant in ministry. They have a hunger and thirst for righteousness, pursuing God's Word and presence daily.
14. Divine destiny and purpose are fulfilled in their lives, and they walk in the fullness of God's plan for them.
15. My children are a light to the world, shining brightly for Jesus and bringing glory to His name.

Chapter 30:

CONCLUSION

As we come to the conclusion of this transformative journey, we are filled with gratitude to the Lord for the opportunity to share our insights from the word of God and experiences with you. Through the power of faith affirmations, we have witnessed miracles unfold, dreams manifest, and lives transformed.

But this is just the beginning.

As you close this book, remember that the power to shape your reality lies within you. Every word you speak, every thought you entertain, has the potential to create the life you desire. Embrace the truth that you are the master of your destiny, and with faith affirmations as your compass, there are no limits to what you can achieve.

We pray that the principles outlined in these pages would serve as a beacon of hope and inspiration as you navigate the journey ahead. Let them remind you of your inherent worth in Christ, your divine purpose, and the limitless potentials that reside within you.

Step out with boldness, courage and unwavering faith, being armed with this new knowledge that you have received from the pages of this book and recreate your world with your faith affirmations. Bring into your world the things that you so desire because you have the power to do so.

Here's to a life filled with abundance, joy, and fulfillment—a life beyond your wildest dreams.

With love and blessings,

The Empyrean Couple

Made in the USA
Monee, IL
04 November 2026

67385768R00046